C000001561

Th

Relaxer

Lynne Robinson, Gordon Thomson & Helge Fisher

PAN BOOKS

First published 1999 by Pan Books

an imprint of Macmillan Publishers Limited
25 Eccleston Place, London SW1W 9NF
and Basingstoke

Associated companies throughout the world

ISBN 0 330 37329 3

9 8 7 6 5 4 3

A CIP catalogue record for this book is available from the British Library.

Text design by Neil Lang
Printed and bound in Belgium

Contents

The Exercises

Introduction

After a long day . . .

Need to unwind after a long day at the office? It's tempting to just collapse in front of the TV, but you will feel far more relaxed and refreshed if you do the following routine instead.

These exercises will calm you and de-stress you – feel the tension around your neck and shoulders melt away. Designed to reverse the effects of being 'hunched over' a desk all day, you will feel lengthened almost as if you've been 'ironed out'. The routine includes relaxation techniques, specific stretches for those muscles which have been held tight, and strengthening exercises for key postural muscles.

Your body has worked hard for you all day. Say 'thank you' and it will repay you one hundredfold tomorrow!

The Eight Principles of the Pilates Method

The exercises in this book have their origins in the work of Joseph Pilates (1880–1967). A well-proven method in existence for over seventy-five years, they also incorporate the latest techniques in both mental and physical training, offering complete body conditioning.

The programme targets the key postural muscles, building strength from within, by stabilizing the torso. The body is gently realigned and reshaped, the muscles balanced, so that the whole body moves efficiently. By bringing together body and mind and heightening body awareness, Pilates literally teaches you to be in control of your body, allowing you to handle stress more effectively and achieve relaxation more easily.

All the exercises are built around the following Eight Principles:

Relaxation	**Co-ordination**
Concentration	**Centring**
Alignment	**Flowing movements**
Breathing	**Stamina**

Before You Begin

▷ All exercises should be done on a padded mat.
▷ Wear something warm and comfortable, allowing free movement.
▷ Barefoot is best, socks otherwise
▷ You may need: a firm flat pillow or folded towel, a larger pillow, a long scarf and a tennis ball.

Please do not exercise if:

▷ You are feeling unwell
▷ You have just eaten a heavy meal
▷ You have a bad hangover or have been drinking alcohol
▷ You have taken painkillers, as it will mask any warning pains

If you are undergoing medical treatment, are pregnant or injured, please consult your medical practitioner. It is always advisable to consult your doctor before taking up a new exercise regime.

Checking Your Alignment

Always take a moment to check that your body is correctly aligned before you start an exercise. Here is a checklist to help . . .

▷ Is my pelvis in neutral? See page 10
▷ Is my spine lengthened, but still with its natural curves? Think of the of the top of the head lengthening away from the tailbone.
▷ Where are my shoulders? Hopefully not up around your ears! Keep the shoulder blades down into your back, a nice big gap between the ears and the shoulders.
▷ Is my neck tense? Keep the neck released and soft. The back of the neck stays long. When lying, you my prefer to place a firm flat pillow under your head so that your chin is parallel to the floor.
▷ Where are my feet? Don't forget them, for if they are misplaced it will affect your knees, hips, and back. Usually, they should be hip-width apart, in parallel. Watch that they do not roll in or out!

The Position of the Pelvis and Spine

If you work with the pelvis and the spine misplaced you run the risk of creating muscle imbalances and stressing the spine itself. You should aim to have your pelvis and spine in their natural neutral positions.

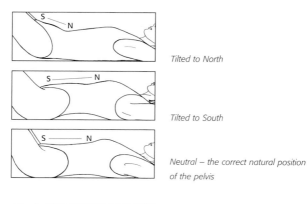

Tilted to North

Tilted to South

Neutral – the correct natural position of the pelvis

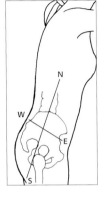
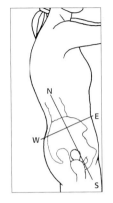
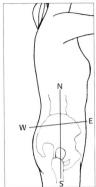

Wrong   *Wrong*   *Right*

Breathing the Pilates Way

In Pilates we use lateral, thoracic breathing for all exercises. This entails breathing into the lower ribcage and back to make maximum use of lung capacity. The increased oxygen intake replenishes the body and the action itself creates greater flexibility in the upper body. It also works the abdominals.

To learn lateral breathing you may sit, stand or kneel, your pelvis in neutral, the spine lengthened.

Wrap a scarf around your ribcage, cross the ends over in the front and pull a little on them to feel where you are working. The idea is to breathe into the scarf, directing the breath into your sides and back, but keeping the shoulders down and relaxed, and the neck calm. The ribs expand as you inhale, close down as you exhale.

Repeat six times but do not over-breathe or you may feel dizzy. Breathe softly in a relaxed way.

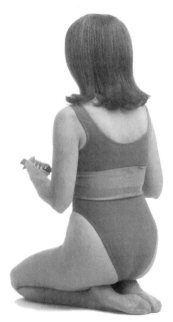

Breathe in wide and full to prepare
*   for movement*
Breathe out as you move
Breathe in to recover

Creating a Strong Centre

Nearly all Pilates exercises involve engaging the deep postural muscles to protect the spine as you exercise. This is called 'stabilizing' or 'centring' and creates a 'girdle of strength' from which to move.

To find these deep muscles, adopt the starting position opposite:

▷ Breathe in to prepare and lengthen through the spine.
▷ Breathe out and engage the muscles of your pelvic floor (as if you are trying not to pass water) and hollow your lower abdominals back to your spine. Do not move the pelvis or spine.
▷ Breathe in and release.

Think of it as an internal zip which begins underneath and zips up and in to hold your lower abdominal contents in place, like zipping up you trousers. '**Zip up and hollow**'.

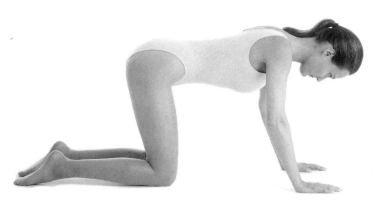

Come onto all fours, hands beneath shoulders, knees beneath your hips. Look straight down at the floor, back of the neck stays long, the spine maintains its natural neutral curve.

The Relaxation Position

Lie with your knees bent. Your feet in line with your hips. Your toes parallel. Your heels in line with the centre of your buttocks. Your chin should be parallel to the floor so place a firm, flat pillow under your head if necessary. Place your hands on your abdomen.

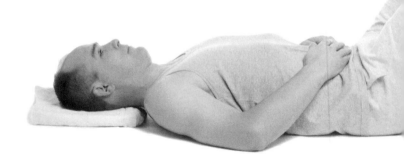

See if you can persuade a friend to read the following instructions, you will have to return the favour of course!

Allow your feet to spread and melt into the floor. Allow the ankles to release. Allow the weight of your legs to transfer into your hip socket and your feet. Release the front of your thighs. Open your hips. Imagine there is sand in your back pockets – let the sand trickle down into the floor. Allow your buttocks to spread. Let your shoulders widen and melt towards the ground. Allow your elbows to open. Imagine your collar bones spreading out like the wings of a bird. Imagine your breast bone softening and gently sinking towards the spine. Be aware of the rise and fall of your abdomen. Notice how every in-breath gently widens your back and how the out-breath contracts the whole rib cage. Allow yourself to be supported by the floor. Release the back of your head into the pillow. Allow your tongue to widen at the base of your mouth. Soften the muscles of your face. Allow the eyes to float in their sockets, the brain to rest in the skull.

Hip Flexor Stretch

This group of muscles get extremely tight when you've been sitting all day.

Starting Position
Lie in the Relaxation position (page 16).

Action
▷ Breathe in wide and full to prepare.
   Breathe out, **zip up and hollow**, keeping that sense of hollow-
   ness in the pelvis, hinge the right knee up to your chest,
   dropping the thigh bone down into the hip joint.

▷ Breathe in as you clasp the right leg below the lower part of the thigh.

▷ Breathe out, still **zipping**, and stretch the left leg along the floor. Your lower back should remain in neutral. If it arches, bend the left knee back up again a little. Hold this stretch for five breaths.

▷ Breathe in as you slide the leg back.

▷ Breathe out, **zip and hollow**, as you lower the right bent knee to the floor, keeping the abdominals engaged.

Repeat twice on each side, keeping your shoulders relaxed and down.

The Hamstring Stretch

Another set of muscles which
are shortened if you sit a lot.

Starting Position

Lie in the Relaxation Position
(page 16). Bring one knee
toward your chest. Holding
a long scarf from underneath,
your palms towards you,
place the scarf over the
sole of one foot. Pelvis
in neutral (page 10).

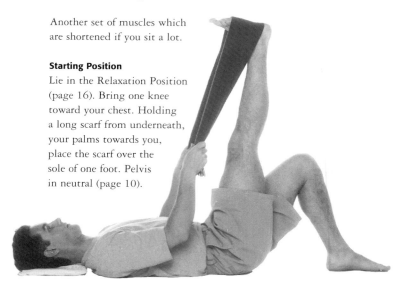

Action

▷ Breathe in wide and full to prepare.

▷ Breathe out, **zip up and hollow**, and slowly straighten the leg into the air. Your pelvis must stay in neutral. Do not allow it to tilt in any direction. If you are comfortable flex the foot down towards your face. Make sure that your leg stays parallel

▷ Breathing normally now, hold the stretch for the count of thirty, before gently releasing it. Keep the tailbone on the floor, lengthening away. Do not overstretch. Keep the upper body open, the elbows soft, the shoulder blades down and the neck long and released!

Repeat three times on each leg.

Shoulder Drops with a Twist

Feel like a massage? This exercise is the next best thing as it loosens the shoulders and releases tension.

Starting Position
Lie with your knees bent. Your feet hip-width apart in parallel. Raise both arms directly above your shoulders with the palms facing inwards.

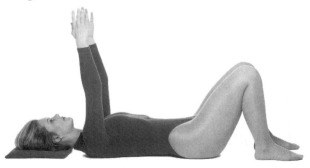

Action

▷ Breathe in wide and full to prepare.

▷ Breathe out, **zip up and hollow**, keeping the pelvis still and square, reach one hand up across the other to where the ceiling meets the wall. Your shoulder blade will leave the floor, your head should move gently with you. Enjoy the stretch between the shoulder blades.

▷ Breathe in and hold the stretch.

▷ Breathe out and relax the shoulder back down to the floor.

Repeat ten times to each side, making sure that the pelvis stays quite still.

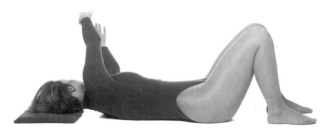

Neck Rolls and Nose Circles

If you suffer from tension headaches, these are for you . . .

Starting Position
Lie in the Relaxation Position (page 16).

Neck Rolls
▷ Slowly and gently allow the weight of the head to roll it to the left.
▷ Return to the centre and over to the right.
▷ Back to the centre and then lift the chin, just a little, to look behind you. Not too far or you'll overarch the neck.

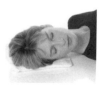
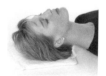
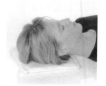

▷ Back to centre and then tuck the chin in, keeping the head on the floor to lengthen the back of the neck.

Repeat the sequence five times.

Nose Circles

Close your eyes. Imagine there is a circle, any size, hovering just above your nose. Slowly draw the circle with your nose, allowing the head to release as you do so. Draw five circles clockwise, five anti-clockwise.

Knee and Leg Circles

To release the muscles around the hip and learn to keep your pelvis stable.

Starting Position
Lie in the Relaxation Position. Wrap a scarf around one thigh, holding it from underneath so that the shoulders stay down and relaxed. Fold the knee up so that it is directly above the hip.

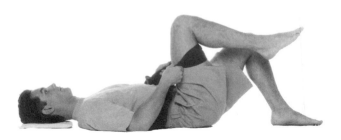

Action

▷ Keeping the pelvis neutral and stable – that is, not allowing it to rock from side to side – gently and slowly circle the bent leg around.

▷ Breathe normally as you do so, **zipping and hollowing** throughout.

▷ Think of releasing the thigh bone from the hip socket. Allow the scarf (and your hands) to help move the leg.

▷ Circle five times clockwise, five anti-clockwise with each leg.

▷ When you have mastered keeping the pelvis still whilst circling the knee, try the exercise without the scarf, then with the leg straight. Keep the upper body open and relaxed and the neck released.

The Diamond Press

A superb exercise for reversing being 'hunched over' all day.

Starting Position
▷ Lie on your front with your feet hip-width apart and
parallel.

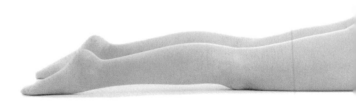

▷ If you have a low back problem, you may wish to place a flat pillow under your stomach.

▷ Create a diamond shape with your arms by placing your fingertips together just above your forehead. Your elbows are open, your shoulder blades relaxed.

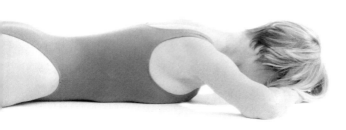

The Rest Position

▷ When you have finished 'The Diamond Press', bring your
  heels together and come back to sit on your heels.* Keep
  the knees apart and take care that you do not sit between
  the heels.
▷ Breathe deeply into the back of your ribcage for eight
  breaths, feel the back expand and contract.
▷ After eight breaths, breathe out, **zip up and hollow**, and
  slowly unfurl the spine, rebuilding the column, vertebra
  by vertebra, until you are upright.
▷ Bring your head up last.

* If you have a knee injury, curl up on your side in the foetal
position.

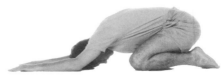

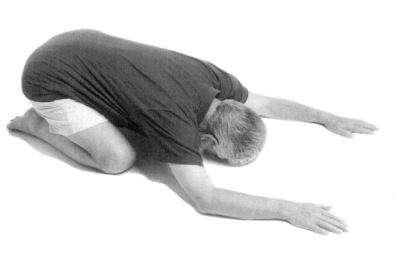

Single Leg Stretch (beginner's)

Starting position

Lie in the Relaxation Position (page 16). Pelvis neutral.

Action

▷ Breathe in wide and full to prepare.

▷ Breathe out, **zipping and hollowing**, and fold one knee at a time onto your chest.

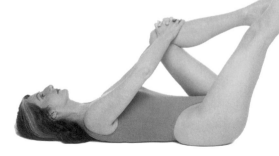

▷ Breathe in and take hold of your left leg with both hands. Keep your elbows open and your breastbone soft. Your shoulder blades stay down into your back. Neck released.

▷ Breathe out, **zip up and hollow**, and slowly straighten the right leg straight up into the air. Keep your back anchored into the floor.

▷ Breathe in and bend the knee back in. Change hands.

Repeat ten times on each leg. Do not allow the leg to fall away from you, your back must stay anchored to the floor. When this becomes easy, you may try the more advanced version overleaf.

Single Leg Stretch (continued)

Action

▷ Breathe in and place the right hand on the outside of the
   right ankle, the left hand on the inside of the right knee.

▷ Breathe out and, **zipping up and hollowing**, slowly stretch
   your left leg away in parallel, so that it is at an angle of
   45 degrees to the floor. The toes are softly pointed.

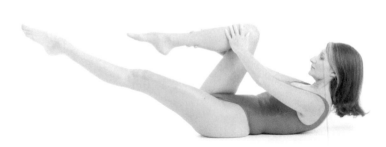

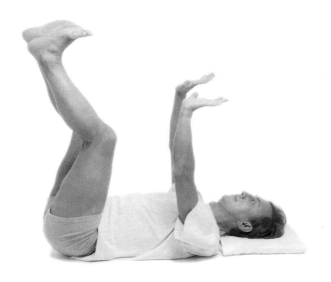

To release the position, bend the knees down onto the chest
before lowering them one at a time. Let your arms cross over
your chest to hug yourself.

Pillow Squeezes

Activate your pelvic floor and work those inner thighs. This exercise also 'opens' the lower back, which is often compressed all day.

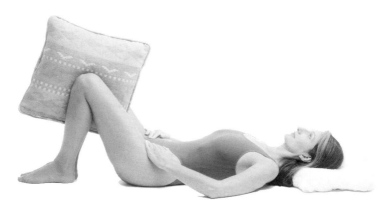

Starting Position

Lie on your back with your knees bent. Place a cushion between your knees. Have your feet together in parallel, your pelvis is in neutral.

Action

▷ Breathe in wide and full to prepare.

▷ Breathe out, **zipping up** the pelvic floor and **hollowing** navel to spine. Squeeze the cushion between the knees. Keep your tailbone on the floor, lengthening away.

▷ Continue to squeeze the cushion for up to ten counts, breathing softly and normally.

Repeat eight times, ensuring that you do not tuck the pelvis, or grip around the hips. Keep your neck and jaw soft and released.

Arm Openings

The ultimate relaxer – we've saved the best till last!

Starting Position
▷ Curl up on your side, with a pillow under your head (a bed
   pillow is ideal). Your back should be in a straight line,
   maintaining its natural curve.

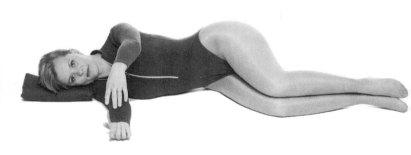

▷ Have your knees bent at a 90-degree angle to your body.
▷ Line all your bones up one on top of the other – your foot
   bones, ankle bones, knees, hips, shoulders.
▷ Stretch your arms out in front of you at shoulder height, the
   palms together.

Please note
Before doing this exercise please consult your practitioner if you
have a disc-related injury.

Arm Openings (continued)

Action

Keep your knees glued together throughout, nailed to the floor, one hip remaining directly over the other, to keep the pelvis in line.

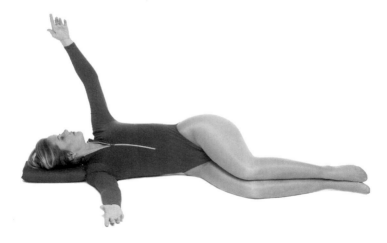

▷ Breathe in, **zip up and hollow**, open your top arm to take
   it behind you, like a door opening. Your eyes follow the
   movement of your arm, so that your head rolls with
   the movement. The elbow stays softly bent, the wrist and
   hand relaxed. The aim is to touch the floor behind you,
   but do not force this or allow the knees to separate.

▷ Breathe out, still **zipping and hollowing**, and slowly bring
   the arm back in a wide arc.

Remember to breathe in as you open breathe out as you close.

Repeat five times, maintaining a strong centre throughout.
Then curl up on the other side and repeat.